CARE OF THE NECK

Second Edition

William K. Ishmael, M.D.

Howard B. Shorbe, M.D.

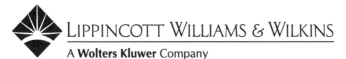

LIPPINCOTT WILLIAMS & WILKINS

A **Wolters Kluwer** Company

Philadelphia · Baltimore · New York · London
Buenos Aires · Hong Kong · Sydney · Tokyo

INTRODUCTION

It is easier to strain the neck than any other part of the body. Strain of the neck can cause painful and uncomfortable aches and "cricks" within the neck itself. It can also contribute to a group of symptoms often called "nervous tension" headache or "cervical tension" syndrome—headaches; dizziness; pain in the face, scalp, and ears; and even feelings of imbalance and "blacking out." One of the most common causes of shoulder and arm pain in people over 40 years old is trouble with the neck.

It is important to realize that severe or chronic pain in the neck can be caused by serious diseases, such as arthritis or osteoporosis, and serious injury, such as a fracture. This booklet deals only with common strain of the neck, which can be treated at home by proper rest, reduction of tension and stress, and improvement of posture. If you experience severe neck pain, or pain or stiffness that does not respond to rest, you should see your doctor.

Remember that some of the worst strains of your neck can occur while you are doing nothing or are sound asleep. Watching television or sleeping in an awkward position can strain your neck as severely as a car accident can. Only proper rest will give relief from strain.

WHY IS THE NECK SO EASY TO STRAIN?

The neck is easy to strain because of the way it is constructed. The neck is made up of seven vertebrae (the "cervical" vertebrae), which

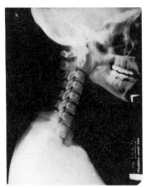

FIGURE 1. The seven vertebrae of the neck. Note forward curve.

are stacked one on top of another. The reason for the potential instability of the neck is shown in the x-ray in Figure 1. As you can see, this stack of vertebrae is actually curved forward when you are in a normal standing position. The vertebrae are supported by muscles and ligaments, linked by small joints called facets, and cushioned by disks of soft cartilage between each vertebra. Consider that this stack of vertebrae and the muscles and ligaments that support it must move almost constantly in all directions as you go about your daily tasks. They must also support the weight of the head, which in the average person is about ten pounds. It is not surprising that your neck is easily strained!

Although a forward curve of the neck is normal, an *excessive* forward curve is likely to lead to a painful strain of the neck, in the same way that an excessive curve can lead to strain in the lower back. In fact, as shown in Figure 2, problems in different areas of the

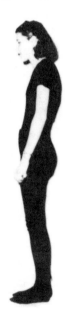

FIGURE 2. Stoop in upper back leads to lower swayback and excessive curvature of the neck.

neck and back may be related and can occur at the same time. A stoop or hunch in the middle of the spine (kyphosis) leads not only to increased sway in the lower back (lordosis), but also to too great a curve in the neck. Clearly, good basic posture will do a great deal to help you avoid both neck and back strain (Fig. 3).

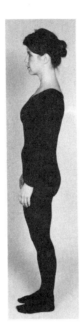

FIGURE 3. Good posture.

If poor posture and excessive curvature are not corrected, they can eventually lead to serious problems. If the head and neck are continually thrust too far forward, it is possible to overstretch the nerve roots that emerge from the cervical spine, which can result in severe neuralgic pain. Degeneration of the cartilage disks between the vertebrae can also compress and interfere with the nerve roots, causing severe pain and disability.

COMMON ACTIVITIES THAT STRAIN THE NECK

Aside from direct injury or diseases such as arthritis or rheumatism, most neck pain is caused by a strain after an unfamiliar exercise or activity, or by holding the neck in an unusual or unnatural position for too long. You are especially prone to neck strain if you lead an inactive life; for example, if you have spent a period of time in bed, your neck structures may easily weaken and become strained when you try to resume normal activities. However, even if you are physically fit and healthy, you can still strain your neck if you force it into an unnatural position for a longer period of time than it can endure.

There are two positions that cause most neck strains:

1. The "forward-thrust" position of the head and neck, which causes excessive curvature of the vertebrae and unusual stress on the neck muscles.
2. Holding the neck rotated or twisted sharply for too long a period of time.

You may find yourself in either of these positions during your most common daily activities. The excessive forward-thrust of the head and neck is also known as the "spectator attitude" because many people fall into the habit of looking sharply upward during activities such as watching a movie or listening to a sermon or speech.

Any task in which your head and neck are extended and bent over your work—such as working at a desk, sewing, knitting, ironing, or talking on the phone—may cause strain to your neck. Bifocal glasses that force you to tilt your head while performing certain tasks can also contribute to neck strain.

Even resting can cause neck strain if you do it in an improper position. Reading while propped in bed, watching television while stretched on a sofa, or sleeping in bed with a pillow that is too high are frequent causes of neck strain. Sleeping in a chair almost always strains the neck and must be avoided at all times. Sleeping with the arms over or under your head can cut off the circulation and can cause tingling, numbness, or pain in the limbs. Also, it causes the head and neck to be propped in an unnatural position. Avoid sleeping positions like this if you can.

Figures 4 through 19 illustrate unnatural body positions that are common causes of neck strain during everyday activities.

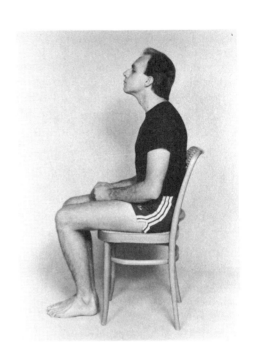

FIGURE 4. Spectator attitude. Don't thrust your neck forward.

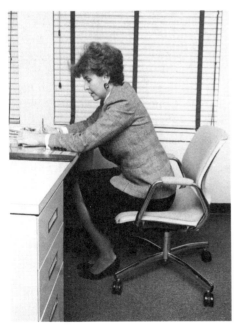

FIGURE 5. Don't lean over your desk.

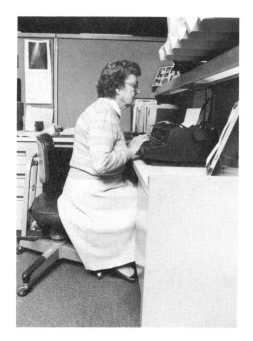

FIGURE 6. Don't sit too far back from a typewriter.

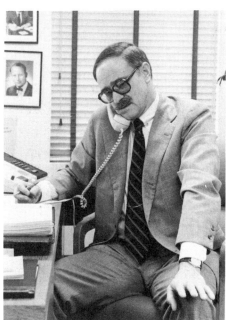

FIGURE 7. Don't twist your neck to hold the phone.

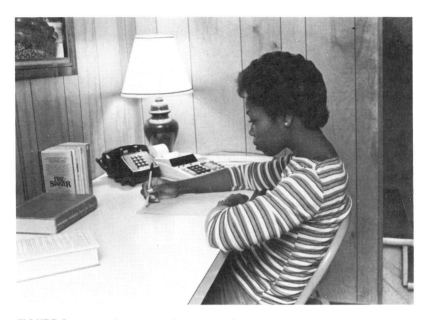

FIGURE 8. Don't lean away from your desk.

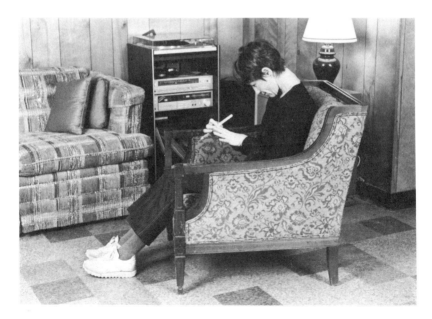

FIGURE 9. Don't lean over your work.

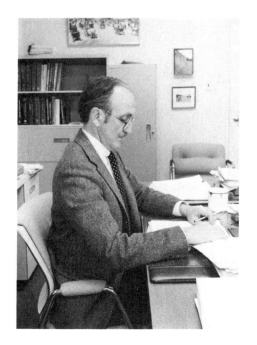

FIGURE 10. If you wear bifocal glasses, don't crane your neck to see.

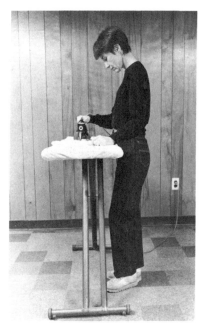

FIGURE 11. Don't bend over an iron.

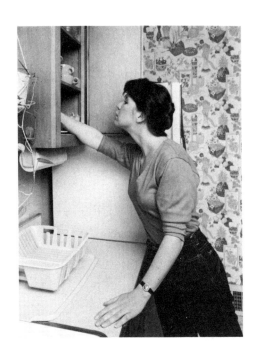

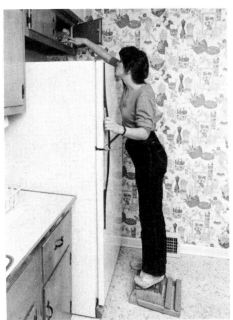

FIGURE 12. (*Top and bottom*) Don't reach up too high.

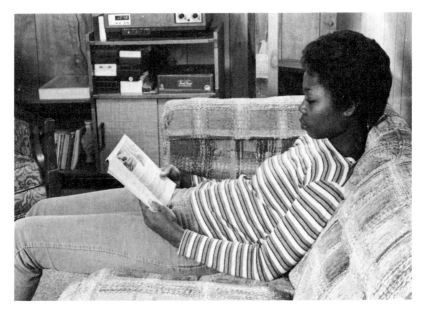

FIGURE 13. Don't slouch on a chair or couch.

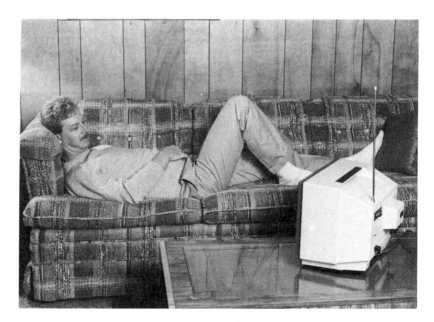

FIGURE 14. Don't lie like this on the sofa.

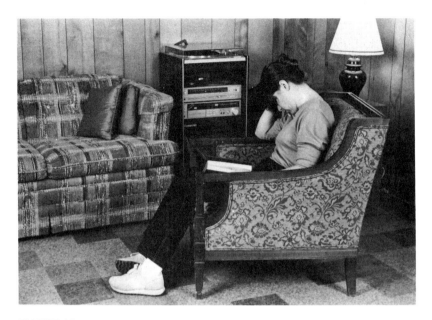

FIGURE 15. Don't sleep in a chair.

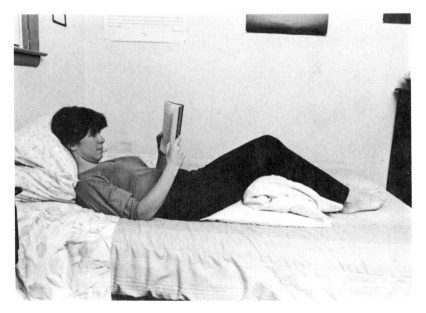

FIGURE 16. Don't read propped up in bed.

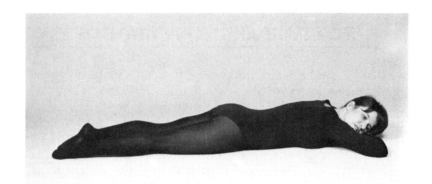

FIGURE 17. Don't sleep on your abdomen.

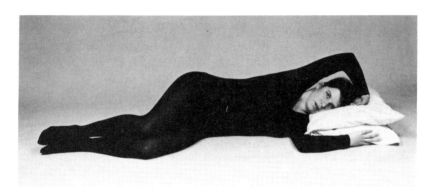

FIGURE 18. Don't sleep with your arm over your face.

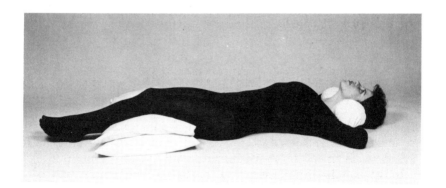

FIGURE 19. Don't lie with your arms behind your head.

NECK PAIN AND YOUR STATE OF MIND

Your state of mind can actually have just as much to do with a pain in your neck as does your physical condition and activity level, and it can be much more difficult to do something about. Tense, high-strung people tend to overexert themselves, thus straining the muscles of the face, head, and neck—this often leads to the well-known "nervous tension" headache. Because no one has a perfect existence completely free of unpleasant situations, everyone suffers from a "nervous tension" headache now and then. Without being aware of it, if you are nervous or tense you can easily twist or bend your neck too far, or for too long a time.

Such people often either work so many hours that they do not get enough sleep or work so hard that they become too tired to go to sleep. It is easy to fall into such a "vicious cycle" of too much work and too little sleep, and the stress that this causes you is very likely to lead to tension and head and neck pains.

If this is a good description of your situation, you will have to do your best to break the pattern. There is little hope that a neck strain will heal until this stress is relieved and time is allowed for proper rest. This may mean slowing your pace or giving up some overtime at work, or having someone else help you with the household chores. It may mean a week of vacation without the children. Only you know what situations contribute most to the tension and strain that affect your neck. But whatever these situations are, try to do something about them, at least for awhile! Your body may be trying to tell you something—your chronic head and neck pain could mean that you have reached your limit for stress.

WHAT TO DO FOR YOUR STRAINED NECK

First, remember that treatment of any neck injury or disorder should be supervised by your doctor. You can do a great deal at home to avoid any further strain on your neck and to strengthen your neck through exercise. But be sure to discuss your recuperation and exercise with your doctor and to obtain your doctor's approval before you begin.

The basic rule for avoiding further neck strain is to keep your neck drawn back and your chin comfortably tucked in, whether you are standing or sitting (Fig. 20). As shown earlier, Figures 5 through 19 illustrate unnatural body positions that strain the neck during everyday activities. Avoid these positions at all times.

Correct

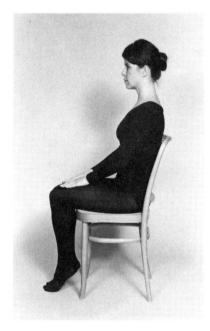

Incorrect

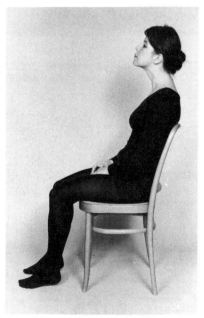

FIGURE 20. Keep your neck drawn back and your chin tucked in.

Here are some tips to follow while your neck strain heals—and afterwards, too:

- Use a chair with arms for support of the back, shoulders, and neck. This will prevent your head and neck from being thrust forward (Fig. 21).

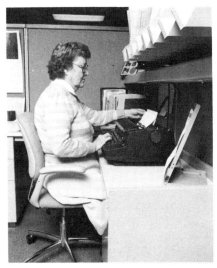

Office

Home

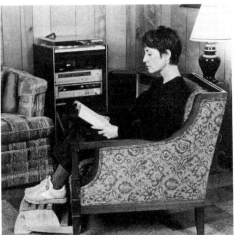

FIGURE 21. Use a chair with arms.

- Make sure your chair is the right height, neither too low nor too high. Sit straight and avoid having to stretch forward or backward while working, eating, and so forth (Fig. 22).

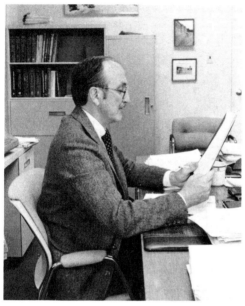

Home

Office

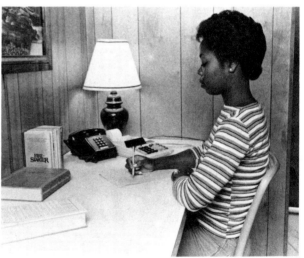

FIGURE 22. Sit straight at your work.

- Make sure your car seat is properly adjusted. If it is too far back or too low, you will need to stretch your neck up and forward to see. Use a pillow, if necessary, to raise yourself to the proper height. Also, a cushion next to you to serve as an "arm" will help support you (Fig. 23).

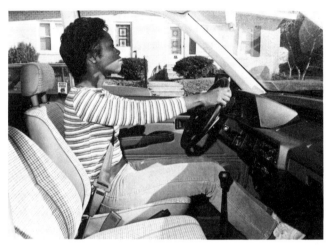

Incorrect

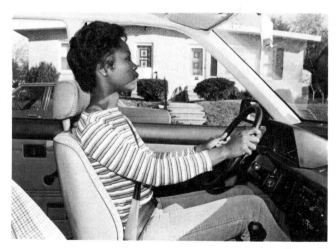

Correct

FIGURE 23. Adjust your car seat properly.

- Do not reach for high shelves, wash windows and so forth, that are higher than your head. Use a stool or a ladder for such activities. Don't reach or look up for any length of time (Fig. 24).

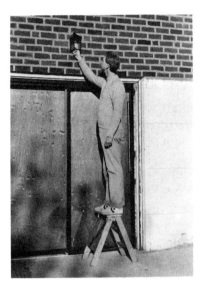

FIGURE 24. Use a stool or ladder when reaching up.

- Avoid sudden, jerky twisting of your head and neck. Slow down and move carefully to avoid strain.
- Never lie on your abdomen or with your head propped forward on high pillows.
- If you sleep on your side, adjust your pillow to maintain your head and neck in a level neutral position. Keep your arms down and your hips and knees bent to avoid neck strain (Fig. 25).

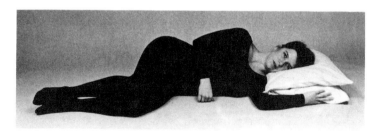

FIGURE 25. Use a pillow to keep your head *level.*

- If you sleep on your back, your pillow should support your head and neck, but it should not force the head forward. A support under your knees will help relax your lower back and will prevent strain (Fig. 26).

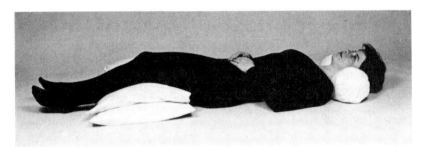

FIGURE 26. The head and neck are supported, not thrust forward.

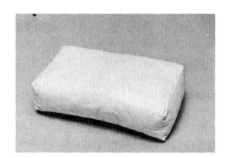

FIGURE 27. Use a good pillow.

- Many people with neck strain simply need to sleep with the proper pillow (Fig. 27). Most people with neck strain should have a pillow 3 or 4 inches thick, 6 or 7 inches wide, and 16 inches long, filled with 4 or 5 layers of Dacron alternated with 8 or 10 layers of crinoline. Two layers of polyurethane foam or sponge rubber may be added for increased firmness in thicker pillows. The pillow should be placed under your *neck*, not under your head, when you sleep on your back. This pillow can be placed on a regular pillow when you sleep on your side. If you cannot find such a pillow, you can have one made for you by an upholsterer.
- Remember, *never* sleep in a chair.

HEAT AND MASSAGE

Applying local heat can often be helpful in reducing the pain of a sore neck. An electric heating pad or a hot water bottle is a common way of applying heat at home. The relief provided by moist heat is often longer-lasting, and at home this can be applied with hot moist towels wrapped in plastic bags to retain the heat. Because many people with neck pain also have painful shoulders or a sore back, it is often helpful to apply heat to all the affected areas together. Applying heat can also help relax your muscles before you perform remedial exercises for a sore back or neck.

Most doctors consider massage a form of therapeutic manipulation, which is, therefore, really effective only when administered by an experienced masseur or physical therapist. However, a simple massage consisting of kneading and stroking of the neck, shoulders, and back is considered beneficial by many people and may be performed by a family member. An increase in pain in any area indicates that the massage is too vigorous or is being done incorrectly.

You may indeed feel relaxed by such a simple massage. If so, that is a very real benefit, and you should certainly make use of it.

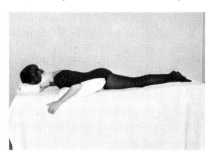

FIGURE 28. Lie in this position for only a few minutes. Note placement of towel and pillow.

Some people with mild, forward-thrust strains of the neck find the position shown in Figure 28 restful. This position is assumed by lying on your abdomen for a short time with a folded towel under your chin or forehead. This will place your neck in a proper "drawn-back with the chin tucked in" position. *This is the only time you should lie on your abdomen.* You should *never* fall asleep in this position or remain in it for more than three to five minutes.

REMEDIAL EXERCISES FOR THE NECK

As mentioned earlier, many people with neck strain also have trouble with the lower back. This is because the neck is part of the spine and, therefore, can be affected by a problem in another area of the spine. If there is an excessive curve in the lower back or a stoop in the middle of the back, the natural curve of the neck also will be affected, most likely becoming excessive (see Figs. 1–4). Consequently, the exercises you do to strengthen and avoid strain to your neck must also strengthen your abdominal muscles, your lower back muscles, and the muscles and ligaments of your upper back and the back and sides of your neck. To avoid further trouble, you must consider your spine as a single unit, limbering up and strengthening all of its muscles and ligaments together.

The following series of exercises is specifically designed to strengthen your neck. (A full series of exercises designed to stretch and strengthen the lower back is described in *Care of the Back*.) If you are recovering from a neck strain or have chronic stiffness and soreness, you should start the exercises slowly and gradually build up your stamina until you can do them three times a day. Mild increased stiffness or soreness during the first few days is to be expected. However, if these exercises continue to cause you increased pain, you should advise your doctor.

Discuss your exercise program with your doctor before you begin doing the exercises, and keep your doctor informed of your progress and of any problems or questions you may have.

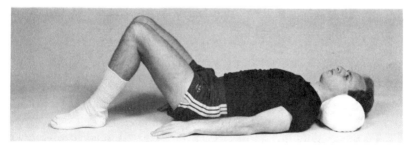

FIGURE 29.   Exercise 1.

Exercise 1 (Fig. 29). Lie on your back with your knees drawn up and your neck supported by a proper pillow. Take a deep breath, expand your chest to its limit, and then exhale slowly. Inhale and exhale very slowly and deeply five or six times. By elevating your ribs, this exercise will help overcome the tendency of an upper back stoop to depress your chest. It will also strengthen your rib muscles. This exercise is particularly helpful when you do it each morning upon awakening.

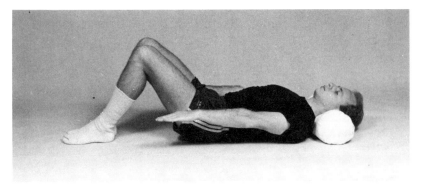

A

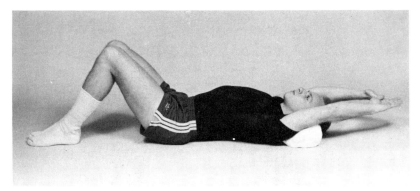

B

FIGURE 30. Exercise 2.

Exercise 2 (Fig. 30A,B). Lie on your back with your knees drawn up and your arms at your sides. Raise your arms six inches and hold them. Then slowly draw your arms back over your head. Touch your hands together, then return your arms to your side. Repeat three to five times, slowly. Note: If you have bursitis or shoulder stiffness, you may find this exercise difficult. If so, perform the exercise cautiously.

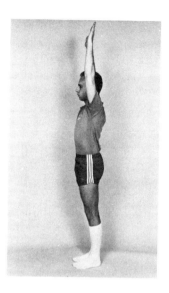

FIGURE 31. Exercise 3.

Exercise 3 (Fig. 31). Lift your arms over your head and stretch them upward. Stand on tiptoe, pull your chin in toward your chest and draw your head backward. Keeping your chin tucked toward your chest, walk on tiptoe several steps.

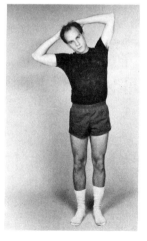
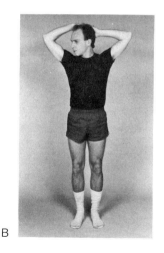

A   B

FIGURE 32. Exercise 4.

Exercise 4 (Fig. 32A,B). While standing, carefully rotate your head in all directions four or five times. If you are recuperating from a neck strain, it is best to delay this exercise until your neck is no longer sore. You should never force the motion in this exercise. You may hear a grinding noise ("crepitation") while performing it. If the noise gets louder, delay the exercise for awhile.

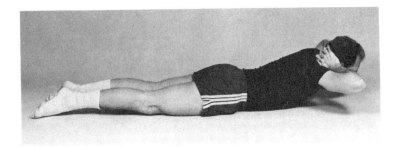

FIGURE 33. Exercise 5.

Exercise 5 (Fig. 33). Lie on your abdomen, with your chin or forehead resting on a folded towel so that your neck is level. Hold your hands on the back of your head, carefully lift your shoulders and head a few inches, and then carefully return to the starting position.

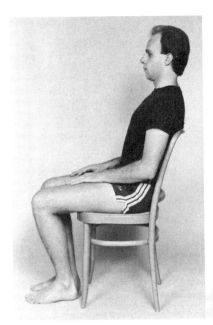

FIGURE 34. Exercise 6.

This exercise is *not* for everyone and should *not* be done if you have any significant neck soreness. If you are not sure whether you should do this exercise, ask your doctor.

Exercise 6 (Fig. 34). You can actually stretch and exercise your neck almost anywhere, at any time of day, whether you are standing or sitting. Simply draw your head back and tuck your chin in toward your chest, then take a deep breath and draw your shoulders back and upward. You should do this exercise several times a day. This exercise is especially good if your work requires you to sit and concentrate for long periods of time, such as working at a desk, or driving.

ISOMETRIC EXERCISES FOR THE NECK

After you have recuperated from a neck strain, it is easy to develop strength in your neck muscles. When your neck muscles are as strong as they should be, they will tend to relax when they should, rather than become stiff and contribute to a headache. A few isometric exercises for the neck, if performed every day, will make a noticeable difference in strength within just a few weeks. If performed faithfully, they will also help slow the sagging of the neck that is part of the process of aging. These exercises can be done in very little time and require no special equipment or expense.

These isometric neck exercises, like all other exercises, should be started gradually. Isometric exercises are deceptively easy but are actually quite strenuous, and they can be overdone in the beginning. At first, it is best to perform each exercise for about one second, at a level just below maximum exertion. From this, you can work up to using full strength and perform the exercises at maximum exertion. Holding an exercise for longer than five seconds will add little to your strength; therefore, if you want to add even more effort, do the exercises several times daily.

While you are learning the exercises, it may be helpful to check your positions by using a mirror. Remember that for maximum benefit, the exercises must be done exactly as illustrated.

A tip in counting off the seconds you hold each exercise—if you say "one hundred and one" at a conversational pace, about one second will pass. If you say "one hundred and one, one hundred and two," about two seconds will pass, and so forth.

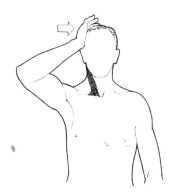

FIGURE 35. Isometric Exercise 1. (Smith C: Isometric Exercises for Men and Women. Philadelphia, JB Lippincott, 1966)

Exercise 1 (Fig. 35). With head held erect and face squarely forward, place the base of the right palm (the part of the palm nearest the forearm) against your head, just above the right ear. Push your head toward the right while resisting with the palm so that there is no appreciable motion. Hold the exercise for the count of "one hundred and one." Repeat this exercise on the left side.

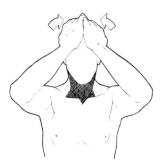

FIGURE 36. Isometric Exercise 2. (Smith C: Isometric Exercises for Men and Women. Philadelphia, JB Lippincott, 1966)

Exercise 2 (Fig. 36). With head held erect and face squarely forward, place the right palm on the right side of your forehead and the left palm on the left side of your forehead, with the hands touching each other. Push your head in a forward direction while resisting with the palms so that there is no appreciable motion. Hold the exercise for the count of "one hundred and one."

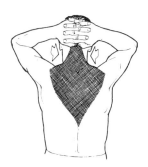

FIGURE 37. Isometric Exercise 3. (Smith C: Isometric Exercises for Men and Women. Philadelphia, JB Lippincott, 1966)

Exercise 3 (Fig. 37). With head held erect and face squarely forward, place the right palm on the right side of the back of the head and the left palm on the left side of the back of the head, intertwining the fingers. Push the head in a backward direction while resisting with the palms so there is no appreciable motion. Hold the exercise for the count of "one hundred and one." Take one or more deep breaths until you are comfortable.

Remember that any general exercise involving the entire body, such as walking, is also good for your neck. Your body will benefit and so will your state of mind, because any exercise that you enjoy can often be the best way to relax yourself mentally as well as physically. This is especially true if you have a confining and exacting job.

So, avoid the painful "spectator attitude" by not being a spectator. Be active and get involved!

SUMMARY

1. Remember that this booklet deals with common strains of the neck, which can be treated by proper rest, by reduction of tension and stress, and by improvement of posture. Severe neck pain or stiffness that does not respond to rest could indicate a serious disease such as arthritis, which requires the immediate attention of your doctor.

2. If you are prone to both neck and back aches, as many people are, you must realize that the problems are related. It is best to exercise and improve the posture of your entire spine as a unit.

3. Do not fall into the habit of sitting with your head and neck thrust too far forward (the "spectator attitude"). Learn to stand and sit properly. This is especially important if your job puts you in a position that causes you to strain your neck all day long, such as working at a desk or table. If this is the case, you must learn to sit properly to avoid strain.

4. You can strain your neck while doing nothing at all. Do not slump or slouch in unnatural positions such as stretching on a sofa watching television or reading while propped in bed. Avoid sleeping on your abdomen at all times.

5. Be sure you are getting enough rest. Stress and tiredness are very frequent causes of neck problems and nervous tension headaches caused by too-tense muscles of the neck and shoulders. Learn to get the rest you need—your body may be trying to tell you something.

6. Use a proper pillow when you sleep, one that does not prop up your head or twist your neck.

7. Never sleep in a chair.

8. Exercise to stretch and strengthen the muscles in your neck. It is impossible to strengthen your neck without exercise.

9. Remember, any general exercise involving the entire body, such as walking, is also good for your neck.

NOTES

NOTES